How I Got Here

My Holistic Healing Journey

by

Darlaina Rose

FOREWORD

We only get one body. So, we're supposed to take care of the one we get. But sometimes, we don't know how.
Darlaina Rose to the rescue. To witness her immense talent and commitment to her gift is nothing short of inspiring. Not only does she have a keen understanding of health and nutrition, but she also shares her knowledge in a way that makes her fans want to learn more.

This book gives people insight into holistic health, by way of Darlaina's experiences. Her transparency would cause anyone to examine their own health choices differently. She opens up about her whole journey and gets to the nucleus of how better decisions can significantly change the outcome.

Darlaina's expertise is rare and the impact that she's made all over the world is indisputable.

Tajuana Ross

#1 Best Selling Author, Award Winning Speaker, Coach

Dedication

I really need to say thank you to my family for all your continued support. To Voncel Harrigan Senior thank you for being the catalyst for all of my creativity. Thank you for everything good, bad and indifferent. What I know for sure is without it there will be no this. Thank you to my parents the late David Martin Senior for always being my dad for making sure that I always have someone to hear me. To my mom Sandra Martin, thank you for being the strongest woman I know. You, raising nine kids (Sharlene, David, Darlaina, Daniel, Deena, Danita, Derrick, Darren and Dianna) well, daddy too. However, you were there day in and day out. We had a good life. Thank you for always supporting me mommy. Thank you for showing us what a wife and mom is, doing so with grace, regardless of what it looks like. Thank you to my brothers and sisters, all 9 of you. I thank you for all your contributions throughout my life. They have pushed me forward. Thank you to my children, (Vontia, Voncel Jr, Vertricia and Vonyel) thank you for being ok with sharing me with the world. Thank you for also being a catalyst for creation. Thank you for all your career and life choices. For all that you continue to do to keep me inspired. To my grandchildren (Vamayah, Viyanah, Vry'Lei, Dhontaye, Dhomontaye, Tahir, Tamir and Tasir) thank you for being a continued gift for all that is to come. It is for your future and my legacy that I work and create, all I do now is for your future. I will leave a legacy for you all.

A special thanks to Bettina. You are the one who sent me down the path of holistic medicine. If it were not for you none of this healing would be happening or have happened. You were truly sent by God that day to save me so that I in return can now save all those lives I now touch.

To My Book Cover Designer C. Montgomery Cooper. Thank you for always being there. No matter what I have ever needed. Logo, marketing material, book covers anything you have been johnny on the spot. Your skills and your eye is perfect. You see the vision the moment I share the thought. You are I true talent. Our friendship is over 30 years old. Thank you for taking this ride with me. Which leads me to the picture you chose on your own without any prompting from me. I am ready for the next cover. You are amazing!

To the most Amazing Photographer Rob Williams. Your eye is a very special gifting. You have the vision before it is even a vision. You shot that photo almost a year ago. Not even for me, for your vision you were working on. You so graciously gave me the shot and C. Montgomery Cooper grabbed it and created this amazing book cover. The eye is truly the window to the soul. I look forward to many more shoots with you.

To all my friends who have contributed time money and energy to any or all my projects here and there, national and international I thank you. You gave me strength and helped me to believe that I could live my life according to my own terms for that I say thank you. There are many of you, but I have to say to Karen, Deidre, Charmar, Glen, Lisa P, Tandra, Vernice, Kemp, Lynn, Jamial, Tracy M, Rochelle, Angel K, Gwen, Dorothy, Serita, Sandi, Kathy R, Jeter, Tejay, Steph, Tariq, Ivy, Nicole B, Lorraine W, Tamara W, Kierra, Toni, Jeanette, Horace, Jones, Sheron, Tierra, Shawn and so many more. Old friends and new friends alike. May my work continue to touch your life in a positive way. I dedicate all the decades of work to all of you who I love and care for so much. Thank you for being there no matter what I am doing. Thank you showing up, contributing and sending me off on whatever journey I was on. Thank you for the 5's, 10's 20's, 50's and 100's. I would not have been here without you. Thank you to my friends who have donated their expertise in systems, photography, graphic design, organization etc. etc. etc. I know for a fact without your services none of my projects would have been realized. THANK YOU ALL!

Note: Darlaina Rose is a Natural Health Professional and her studies have included body systems, Herbs and natural nutrition. As a Natural Health Professional, she teaches about natural health maintenance giving clients consultations pertaining to the natural means by which they can have a healthier lifestyle. She deals strictly in helping people to improve their general health and fitness through better nutrition; improved lifestyle and health habits; and positive mental attitudes. Darlaina Rose is NOT a Medical Doctor and cannot legally diagnose diseases, prescribe drugs or recommend treatments for specific disease conditions and that she will not perform any functions of a licenses field.

TABLE OF CONTENTS

The Beginning of the Beginning

It was a regular ol' workday. Full of all the usual stresses. Working in a hospital Business office has always full of drama. My boss was amazing though. Ms. Scott was a mom's mom. She took care of the staff. So, the day that I felt like my arm was numb. I told her I felt weird. She told me to go to the ER. Here I am at a hospital, a long term acute care facility. NO ER. So, I promised I would go after work. Not only did I go after work, but I caught the bus and the subway to get there. DON'T DO THAT!!

All I can say is that if you feel any of the following symptoms don't wait, don't hesitate!!

- Arm Numbness, Weakness

- Nausea

- Vomiting

- Heart palpitations (a sudden pounding, fluttering, or racing feeling in the heart)

- Lack of energy

- Dizziness (feeling faint or light-headed)

- Chest discomfort (pain, pressure, or discomfort in the chest)

- Shortness of breath (difficulty breathing during normal activities)

Or no symptoms at all!

Well I arrived at Temple University and, so it began, Darlaina the heart patient! Did she have a heart attack? we think you had a mild heart attack!! Whaaattt! For now take this aspirin and we are going to give some fluids and run some test. Oh yes, I was admitted to the hospital and down the rabbit whole I went. Into a world of illness that included medication and a lot of DOCTORS!!! I'm not sick I thought I have never been sick this has got to be an error. I just need to rest more, I mean work is a little stressful. Hospital Accounts Receivables, can get real. It was crazy when the hospital CFO began calling me directly. Did we get the Blue Cross money yet Darlaina? That could rattle anyone feathers. He was, well, still is a very nice guy. He didn't know he was freaking me out. Did my body respond in this negative way because of stress? I mean I know they say stress kills but REALLY!! This was bad, and I was afraid. I'm still young, well to me I was young. Am I going to die? I have children and grandchildren now. I can't die! Lord please help me! After 2 days, Darlaina you have congestive heart failure. Your heart doesn't pump like everyone else's. You heart is weak. It is pumping at 35% capacity. We are going to connect you to a Holter monitor. This will monitor over the next 24-48 hrs.

A Holter monitor is a battery-operated portable device that measures and records your heart's activity (ECG) continuously for 24 to 48 hours or longer depending on the type of monitoring used. The device is the size of a small camera. It has wires with silver dollar-sized electrodes that attach to your skin.

I am in here and being tested every which way. It is crazy!! They are acting like my days are numbered. The word goes out to the family. One by one they find their way to me. Telling me not to worry all will be ok. It is finally decided after a week in the hospital that I can go home on meds. Medicine ok, I can work with that. The first prescription was for Cozaar, this is for what doc? Cozaar (losartan) is an angiotensin II receptor antagonist. Losartan keeps blood vessels from narrowing, which lowers blood pressure and improves blood flow. Cozaar is used to treat high blood pressure (hypertension) in adults and children who are at least 6 years old. They didn't tell me about the blood pressure part. Just it keeps the blood vessels from narrowing. This is the list that I found in my research of the side effects. I never looked or even asked about the side effects at the time. I amazed at all this stuff.

•Abdominal or stomach pain

•anxiety

•bladder pain

•bloody or cloudy urine

•blurred vision

•chills

•cold sweats

•coma

•confusion

•cool, pale skin

•depression

•difficult breathing

•difficult, burning, or painful urination

•dizziness

- fast heartbeat

- frequent urge to urinate

- headache

- increased hunger

- irregular heartbeat

- lower back or side pain

- nausea or vomiting

- nightmares

- numbness or tingling in the hands, feet, or lips

- pale skin

- seizures

- shakiness

- shortness of breath

- slurred speech

- troubled breathing with exertion

- unusual bleeding or bruising

- unusual tiredness or weakness

- weakness or heaviness of the legs

•Arm, back, or jaw pain

•chest pain or discomfort

•chest tightness or heaviness

•dizziness, faintness, or lightheadedness when getting up suddenly from a lying or sitting position

•fainting

•fast, irregular, pounding, or racing heartbeat or pulse

•inability to speak

•pain or discomfort in the arms, jaw, back, or neck

•severe or sudden headache

•sweating

•swelling or puffiness of the face

•temporary blindness

•unsteadiness or awkwardness

•weakness in the arm or leg on one side of the body, sudden and severe

•weakness in the arms, hands, legs, or feet

Incidence not known •Black, tarry stools

•bleeding gums

•cough

•dark urine

•difficulty with swallowing

•general tiredness and weakness

•hives

•itching

•large, hive-like swelling on the face, eyelids, lips, tongue, throat, hands, legs, feet, or sex organs

•light-colored stools

•muscle cramps or spasms

•muscle pain or stiffness

•pinpoint red spots on the skin

•puffiness or swelling of the eyelids or around the eyes, face, lips, or tongue

•skin rash

•upper right abdominal or stomach pain

•yellow eyes and skin

Some side effects of losartan may occur that usually do not need medical attention. These side effects may go away during treatment as your body adjusts to the medicine. Also, your health care professional may be able to tell you about ways to prevent or reduce some of these side effects. Check with your health care professional if any of the following side effects continue or are bothersome or if you have any questions about them.

More common

•visual disturbance

•body aches or pain

•decreased vision

•dry cough—THIS WAS THE ONE, HAD ME SOUNDING LIKE AN OLD MAN. I went to the doctor told her that I thought I was coming down with the flu. She chuckled and said, "oh no Darlaina that's a side effect of the medication." Whaaat!! She said that I didn't have to worry because she said that she could give me a medicine for that. I said oh no, you want to give me a medicine for my medicine. No ma'am why can't we just change it to something else. She did but I don't know what. It's all a blur. A memory my brain has chosen not to have. These memories no longer serve my greater good.

Now carry on with the side effects:

•ear congestion

•loss of voice

•nasal congestion

•runny nose

•sneezing

•sore throat

Less common

•Acid or sour stomach

•back pain

•belching

•difficulty with moving

•heartburn

•increased sensitivity to pain

•increased sensitivity to touch

•indigestion

•joint pain

•lack or loss of strength

•pain in the knees or legs

•pain or tenderness around the eyes and cheekbones

•stomach discomfort or upset

•swollen joints

•trouble sleeping

•weight gain

Rare

•Ankle, knee, or great toe joint pain

•bloated

•change or loss of taste

•depression

•difficulty having a bowel movement (stool)

•dry skin

•excess air or gas in the stomach or intestines

•full feeling

•hair loss or thinning of the hair

•hearing loss

•increased sensitivity of the skin to sunlight

•loss of appetite

•passing gas

•redness or other discoloration of the skin

•severe sunburn

AND THAT'S ONLY ONE MEDICATION! As I am looking at them now. I am noticing that I had additional side effects but just didn't know that they were side effects. SMH

2 SIDE EFFECTS:

Diovan

GENERIC NAME(S): Valsartan is used to treat high blood pressure and heart failure. It is also used to improve the chance of living longer after a heart attack. In people with heart failure, it may also lower the chance of having to go to the hospital for heart failure. Valsartan belongs to a class of drugs called angiotensin receptor blockers (ARBs). It works by relaxing blood vessels so that blood can flow more easily. Lowering high blood pressure helps prevent strokes, heart attacks, and kidney problems.

Dizziness or lightheadedness may occur as your body adjusts to the medication. If any of these effects last or get worse, tell your doctor or pharmacist promptly.

To reduce the risk of dizziness and lightheadedness, get up slowly when rising from a sitting or lying position. Tell your doctor right away if you have any serious side effects, including: fainting, symptoms of a high potassium blood level (such as muscle weakness, slow/irregular heartbeat).

Although valsartan may be used to prevent kidney problems or treat people who have kidney problems, it may also rarely cause serious kidney problems or make them worse. Your doctor will check your kidney function while you are taking valsartan. Tell your doctor right away if you have any signs of kidney problems such as a change in the amount of urine.

A very serious allergic reaction to this drug is rare. However, get medical help right away if you notice any symptoms of a serious allergic reaction, including: rash, itching/swelling (especially of the face/tongue/throat), severe dizziness, trouble breathing.

Common side effects of Diovan:

Abnormally Low Blood Pressure Severe

High Amount of Potassium in The Blood Severe

Backache Less Severe

Diarrhea Less Severe

Dizzy Less Severe

Head Pain Less Severe

Infection Caused by A Virus   Less Severe

Intense Abdominal Pain   Less Severe

Joint Pain   Less Severe

Low Energy   Less Severe

Infrequent side effects of Diovan:

Kidney Disease with Reduction in Kidney Function Severe

Acute Infection of The Nose, Throat or Sinus Less Severe

Blood Pressure Drop Upon Standing Less Severe

Cough Less Severe

Feel Like Throwing Up Less Severe

Inability to Have an Erection Less Severe (less severe, by whose interpretation!)

Throwing Up Less Severe

Rare side effects of Diovan:

Abnormal Liver Function Tests Severe

Blurred Vision Severe

Chest Pain Severe

Decreased Blood Platelets Severe

Decreased Neutrophils a Type of White Blood Cell Severe

Feeling Faint Severe

Giant Hives Severe

Hepatitis Severe

Inflammation of the Skin with Blisters Severe

Rhabdomyolysis Severe

Trouble Breathing Severe

Vasculitis Severe

Chronic Trouble Sleeping Less Severe

Constipation Less Severe

Cramps Less Severe

Drowsiness Less Severe

Dry Mouth Less Severe

Feeling Anxious Less Severe

Feeling Weak Less Severe

Gas Less Severe

Hair Loss Less Severe

Heart Throbbing or Pounding Less Severe

Indigestion Less Severe

Itching Less Severe

Loss of Appetite Less Severe

Muscle Pain Less Severe

Numbness and Tingling Less Severe

Rash Less Severe

Sensation of Spinning or Whirling Less Severe

Throat Irritation Less Severe

I remember one of the pills being a water pill or diuretic. Diuretics. Often called water pills, diuretics make you urinate more frequently and keep fluid from collecting in your body. Diuretics, such as furosemide (Lasix), also decrease fluid in your lungs so you can breathe more easily.

Because diuretics make your body lose potassium and magnesium, your doctor also may prescribe supplements of these minerals. If you're taking a diuretic, your doctor will likely monitor levels of potassium and magnesium in your blood through regular blood tests. I didn't even know that I needed my potassium and magnesium monitored. I was in the dark about most of my treatment. I did whatever they told me I had to do.

The Psychiatric drug! ----whaaaatttt the fat world? As my brother would say. My cardiologist said, I want to try a drug that has been known to help. It is a psych drug though. I said ok I will try it. I didn't want it to ruin my event packed weekend and decided to take it on Sunday evening. All I know is I immediately became sleepy. I laid down and the hallucinations began. There were people all over my bedroom. They were looking at me, I was afraid, so I ducked my head under the covers and guess what? They were there too! I was screaming, saying to the people GET OUT OF HERE! When I called out of work and went back to the doctor. He wanted me to stay on it. I refused and asked what or who could possibly need that. I was unable to work. Any imaginary friend I had ever had in my life was there, right in front of my eyes. It was scary. I saw things that weren't there. I never took one more tablet of that. I have no time not to be in control of my mental faculties. Here's the real question: why give that to someone without mental illness especially if there are other options? Whose idea was that? Drug companies maybe? Who knows but it was not for me!! DEEE-CLLINNEEE!   They would try different medications sometimes I could tell my medications were going to change because I saw a pharmaceutical marketing representative was at my doctor's office. This is with most chronic or terminal illness. Hopefully the medication won't kill you before the disease does.

Our family friend was diagnosed with pancreatic cancer. It was devastating to him and his family. He started treatment. He died of a heart attack. That made no sense he didn't have a bad heart. Guess what it was a side effect of one of the chemotherapy drugs. His son found him, now that is his son's story. Very sad. What would make someone take a drug that the side effect is a heart attack? What did they tell him? Did they tell him? Did he read the medicine insert? Did he know? We don't know? What we do know is he didn't die of cancer.

Darlaina Rose the heart patient.

I would now have to follow up with a cardiologist from now on. OMG! I go home with I don't know how many meds, told to rest and that I could do nothing stressful. I am not even allowed to drive!! No Road Rage for me I guess. Take this one 3x a day with food, take this one 2 x a day on an empty stomach. Make sure you watch out for that long list side effects.

HEART FAILURE AND TRANSPLANT UNIT

I've been home from the hospital a week or so and now it is the today, this is the day I go see the cardiologist. I arrive at the HEART FAILURE AND TRANSPLANT UNIT, that's the name! Talk about the power of words. Everyone in there looked sick. I'm not sick as them. My heart is going to get better. Why do they call it the Heart Failure and Transplant Unit? Don't they realize the power of words and vision. Now every time I walk into this place I am affirming heart failure and the vision of a possible heart transplant every single time!

This is not good at all. I continue to go monthly it seems. It is a real rabbit hole. Once you go in its hard to get out.

You can get so far in that you don't come out alive. They ushered me into the exam room and I wait a few minutes for the doctor. When she finally walked in, she walked right back out. I sat there looking puzzled what was that about. Then she came back in and said I'm looking for Darlaina the heart patient. I said yes, that's me. She said my goodness you are not text book at all. You are not overweight, not one other indicator for heart disease. I agreed but there I was a patient at the Heart Failure and Transplant Unit. Down the rabbit hole I go.

MIND BODY AND SOUL

We are connected mind, body and soul. According to Louise Hay diseases of the heart come from heartbreak. I was having some major marital problems during that time. That made sense. It made sense because I had no markers for heart disease at all. After reading You can heal your life by Louise Hay. I understood how I acquired my heart problems.

Prior to one of my visits to the cardiologist I had a nasty cough. I mean nasty, I mean that if you heard it you moved your seat nasty. It hurt when I coughed. I arrived at the cardiologist office for my regular visit.

THE HEART FAILURE AND TRANSPLANT UNIT!

As soon as she comes in I tell her about my cough and that I surely was coming down with something. She chuckled and said 'oh no Darlaina that is a side effect of the medication. Its ok, though, I can give you something for that". Another medicine, I asked? She said yes. Well I said No! Absolutely not! A medicine for my medicine that made no sense to me. Why don't we take me off this one and get another one without the cough side effect? She complied with my request. Another reminder of our dear family friend again who was diagnosed with pancreatic cancer. He died of a heart attack! A side effect of the cancer drug. I think sometimes when we read these side effects we like to believe that it would never happen to you. That we are somehow immune to the bad stuff. I have watched many of my friends and family lose their lives over chronic illness and disease.

Bettina Said it……

I, for a while thought that that would be my fate until…. In walks Bettina, my friend, leaner than I remember. It had been some time maybe more than a year or more since I saw her. She said to me as I lay on my sofa. "Darlaina you have to take control of your own health. Those doctors are going to kill you". Not on purpose of course, but eventually the body will give out. I have learned now that when the body is inundated with toxins something will break down. System after system.

I was sooooo tired as she was speaking. She said you just must, doctors mean well but we are all not the same. We are not textbook.

The Journey Begins

During her visit Bettina suggested I read "the Secret "I said ok I would

17

check it out, but I was very nonchalant about it or really just too tired to hear. I was living the best I could trying to care for my family and work. I had more days out of work than in. I was in and out of the hospital. I finally got a copy of the Secret on DVD. I watched it. I was shocked. People in the movie were healing themselves with their thoughts! They were using herbs. Interesting concepts I thought. I am going to be more prayerful and I'm not going to think about dying anymore. I'm not going to talk about being sick and possibly dying anymore. I was resolved. As resolved as I was it didn't stop me from getting ill. I had gotten the flu, I was so congested I could barely breathe. One of the ladies from our congregation suggested that I go to see Dr. Wyatt. I only agreed because I was so messed up. She took me there. It was a little rinky dink store front located at 40th and walnut sts in Philadelphia, pa. In my head I was thinking I don't know exactly what they do here, but they need to dust or something. There were bottles of herbs, tinctures and teas on all four walls. There were 4 metal folding chairs in the middle of the floor. "The waiting room". So, I waited. Finally, they call me up. This was not Dr Wyatt. This was some young guy. Hi name was Diego. He greeted me than started to wave his hand around my head. While he was waving one hand the other hand was on his side and one finger was moving back and forth it was very umm weird. As he waved his hand over my head, he said you have a bunch of male stress that's your husband, then he waved on the other side and said that's more male stress that's your son. I said hold up wait a minute!!! I AM A CHRISTIAN, I DON'T DO VOODOO! I was afraid! He said oh no ma'am! We practice Kinesiology the study of the body's energy. Oh, I said, whew! I surely was about to high tail it out of there. He continued.... Left side male stress, husband, right side male stress son. There is a heart issue what's wrong with your heart? Oh no don't tell me. He continues, lactose intolerance, hip injury, knee injury and bunion on your foot. All accurate!!! He began pulling down herbs and tinctures just for me. He had them all on the counter. He asked for my hand, placed it on top of all the herbs he had for me. I asked why? He said that everything is energy. He placed my hand on top of all the herbs he had on the counter. He then placed his hand on top of mine. He shook his head no, and exchanged a few of them out. He placed my hand again on top and then his and he said, "yes we got it now." He pulled out a legal paid and began writing. He wrote take this 3x a day, that 2x etc. etc. He added drink 8 glasses of water per day, exercise for 15 min a day and said that I would live a long time. I went home with $114.00 worth of herbs and instructions written on a legal pad with the prescribed dosages by Diego.

Oh! my goodness what am I doing? Will this work? Am I crazy? Is this quackery? I don't know but I'm going to try it. I started taking the herbs, exercising and drinking water. When I say exercising I mean just walking a little up and down my stairs at home. I was in no way ready for the exertion of real heart pumping exercise. I changed my diet to all natural and organic. I knew the sodium content for everything that I ate. My children used to get upset because I knew the sodium content of everything they ate. I would say things like, don't eat that biscuits they have 500 mg of sodium I would say. I didn't even keep salt in the house. I began to buy things like organic fruits and vegetables, grass fed chicken, organic salad dressing. I ate more whole foods one ingredient foods like oranges, bananas, apples etc. It was different. If food was overcooked, wilted. I knew that all the nutrients were in the pot. I usually did not eat it. I would find more colorful vibrant food. Food for me had to look happy. Even if I went to a restaurant if the food didn't look as good as the picture. I sent it back. My food had to look happy to make me happy. That is still true to this day. I was learning all there was about food and herbs.

On the Right track

Finally, feeling better I can go out in the cold, I can go out in the heat. I'm not as winded when I walk the stairs. I'm getting better. My diet is good, I'm exercising well walking my stairs in my house. I'm drinking my 8 glasses of water daily. I am doing really good. I'm reading and listening to positive mental attitude things. Personal development, I loved what I was reading and hearing from Oprah, Dr Phil, Lisa Nichols, Jack Canfield, John Asaraf, Bob Proctor and so many more. My mind was expanding. I was getting better, mind body and soul. I learned how to find great versions of the herbs. I learned they can be purchased at highs and lows. No matter the budget you can find a great starting place. The food was interesting too! The flavors where SOOO vibrant. The food tasted better. I was getting back to normal all was well.

Time to Tell

Finally, I had weaned myself off all the drugs. (NOTE: DON'T DO THAT, I COULD HAVE KILLED MYSELF FOR REAL WEANING MYSELF OFF THOSE DRUGS)

I was 100% using herbs for my heart. I felt better than I ever had. I had energy, not winded when walking stairs. Its' time to say something. It has been 5 months. I go to my sister Sharlene's office and told her that I was off all meds. She was like whaaat! You have a heart condition you have to take the meds. I said no I feel amazing. She was not having any of that. She told me that if I didn't go to the doctor she would call my mommy! Nooooo, okaaayyyy! I will go to the doctor.

20

I went to my primary doctor a few days later. I thought he was going to say how good it was that I had not been hospitalized for a while. As soon as he got wind that I was no longer taking my medications he hit the ceiling! No way, Kathy get to the back and give me a sample of some drug he had back there. I said nope I feel great! He fussed at me for a bit, then he said that if I wasn't going to take the medicine that I would need to see the cardiologist the same day. He scolded me so bad! You have got to go TODAY DARLAINA! He called my husband and told him I needed to go to the cardiologist right away. He really called and told on me. So, my husband arrived at the doctor's office in a hurry. He was trying to figure out what all the hub bub was about. Parks explained that I was not on the medications I was subscribed. I'm almost certain he knew but you know men don't really pay attention like that. Only when necessary. Too funny, right? So off I went, we went. When we arrived, the cardiologist examined me. He was not my original cardiologist. He kind of side-eye me too, congestive heart failure? Really?

He told me that I didn't seem to be in any distress. He said he would not at this point put me on medication. He said because he has patients that need to be off medicine but refuse to stop taking the medications. However, he said that he wanted to run some test and that depending on the results if I needed to be on prescription therapy, he wanted to me to be open to that. I agreed, with my head hung down low. I knew that I didn't want to take anymore drugs.

Testing Begins

I had all kinds of testing over 3 weeks. Ekg, stress test, cardiac catherization, etc. All the results were gathered, and he called me in to discuss the results. He showed me 3D pictures and videos of my heart. They were colorful and detailed. I thought I have the bomb dot com insurance because they paid for some pretty spectacular test. He pointed out some things. He said something about electricity is what I remembered.

Then he said it! Those words that would change the trajectory of my life. He said I don't know what they told you had, but, I can't find anything wrong with your heart.

Whaaaaaattttt!!! I'm healed!! Oh! let the happy dance begin. I mean I knew I was feeling better. But wow! Wow! Wow! 5 months to the day my heart was completely healed. Wow Wow Wow!!! It worked! It all worked. It was not easy, but I did it! With a lot of prayer and support its done! Hallelujah!!

Darlaina Rose is healed, she is no longer a heart patient. Well on paper I will always be but in real life NOPE! I continue to live this all natural and organic life. I share my story repeated. Help as many people as I can by sharing this story. I decided that I loved helping people and enrolled in Institute for Professional Excellence in Coaching. It was amazing, I went from girrrrrl if that was me, to how does that make you feel? And what would be better for you? I evolved from being just that shoulder to cry on to someone effecting real change in others' lives, on a small scale. I had a few speaking engagements too! I found out I loved speaking and helping people.

You Quit, but I don't?!

It has been an amazing few years health wise. However, my family is changing. My family is changing. My marriage is dissolving. My husband of 27 years has asked for a divorce. He said he just didn't want to do it anymore. We were married very young 17 and 18. We really didn't any young adulthood. He had had his first child at 15. Now we are married. Chile, we ain't know what we were doing. Married at 18, first child at 19 no I wasn't pregnant when we got married but we wasted no time. Married ok baby next right yup! Don't do that! Get to know who you married before you bring babies in the mix. We keep going second baby 21. It was a lot. I didn't understand but, I oblige him. Oh! my Goodness, my marriage is over. How will I get through this one?! This is my life it is all I have ever known. Sure, we had problems, we've been through all the bad stuff. Why now, all is quiet. I don't understand but, ok. I was sick to my stomach, I was hurt. I was suicidal, I was homicidal. I was going to kill him, kill me, kill the dog!! I don't know but someone was going to get it! It's funny now but it sure was not funny then. Our marital home was a huge 3-story home. It was expensive to care for. I decided it would be best for me to get a smaller home for me and my young daughter. I did it! I bought a house all by myself. Well with the help of my amazing girlfriend Con and a mean real estate agent Lisa. What an accomplishment! Many thanks to the hard work of my good friend Connie. I used my skills of Lisa. I was buying a lot of used furniture. I actually placed an ad in craigslist for help. I wonder if its archived. Let me check! Hold on a second ……

Craigslist Ad: Don't Throw it away! Give it to me. *Recently separated single mother of 13 yr. old girl. Need home furnishing, dishes, linens, beds etc. will pick up.* I did that too! I traveled to Coatesville for dishes, Broomall for kitchen set, somewhere for the microwave, a bedroom set, man, what a journey? Most of the items were either free or very low fees. It used to be a joke people asking me what I got from craigslist and the prices. It was unbelievable. Between craigslist, the flea market and the thrift store my house became a home. Unless I shared that information, no one knew how I did it. I used to tour people around my entire house and show them what I got from craigslist or the thrift store. I was clean, nice and stylish.

THE BOOK – The Gurlz are Born

Then it happened I received a book. I'm not sure how I got it from that day to this, but I got it! It saved me!! I was reading it and crying and crying and reading and it hit me! Hard! I can't be the only one, why not cry together?! I started the No Matter What Book Group. Named after Lisa Nichols Book, No Matter What! 9 steps to living the life of your dreams. Oh! how this book changed my life and the lives of the women I shared it with. Amazing Amazing! We met every Tuesday at 630 and we went over the chapters and the exercises. We wrote love letters to ourselves, we told the truth out loud! It was soooooo good and Juicy as Lisa would say. We were growing together. All of us. I facilitated but I was growing too! The group was growing too! 4, 8, 10 uh oh we are growing. We were truly getting to the nitty gritty of what was going on in the lives of the women who attended. We were tackling relationships, self-esteem, self-love, relationships, career choices, business idea and so much more. There were many lives changed in that group. It grew and grew. It was so much fun to meet with the ladies' week after week. We never knew if we would get through a chapter because we allowed each other to share what was on your heart. If something was going on it was a NO JUDGEMENT SAVE SPACE. Here you could lay your heart down and it would be cared for. You could cry, scream, cuss whatever and we supported our member. POINT BLANK PERIOD. We continued to grow moved out of my home and moved to a store front. The Vendors Boutique. We needed space to spread out. Lisa welcomed us with open arms. We were growing. It was an amazing place to be. Every Tuesday at 6:30 we were there. We were changing our lives together. It was an experience that I would never change. It was us, **Just the Gurlz!** We were and still are a women's empowerment community. Any woman can walk into our session a stranger and leave a part of the family. We were a real community. Just the Gurlz – was born. The name was changed. We were off to the races. We believed that all women should be able to stand on her own financial, spiritual and emotional feet and we were going to learn how to do it together.

A special thanks to Bettina. You are the one who sent me down the path of holistic medicine. If it were not for you none of this healing would be happening or have happened. You were truly sent by God that day to save me so that I in return can now save all those live I know touch.

Announcement

I am happy to announce the Re-Launch of Just The Gurlz – Women's Empowerment Community In Philadelphia, Pa Scheduled for March 2018. Just in time for Women's Month. I hope to see you there. *Ambassadors Always Needed.* Become and ambassador and help me spread the word that We as women can do anything! Whatever you set your heart to do is already done. I have great goodies for ambassadors too. Let's have some fun and change lives together.

Settling into Single

I was settling in to being single again. I wasn't liking it, but it was my reality. I mean how long was I single. I was married at 18. I had no idea what it meant to be single, but I was ready to find out. So, I thought anyway. In my own home, learning how to live on my own. I was learning how to sleep alone. That was hard. I was learning who I was and what I wanted in my life. I was now learning how to live on my terms. That was such a transition. Transition to taking care of only me. I forgot to eat especially when my daughter wasn't home. I had no one to cook for. Yup to me I was nobody. I prepared for my women's group weekly. I had hand outs and gratitude rocks. I was pouring into the women all that I had. I wanted them to be well and live well. I tried very hard to stay spiritually grounded. I prayed a lot. I asked God why? That answer would come much later.

I worked and served everybody I could. That kept the hurt away. My children, my grands, my co-workers whoever needed me. Then, a family situation came up and I became a foster mother. I had been raising other people children my whole life anyway. It became a joke between my friends. They would say if I ever didn't want my kids I'm dropping them off to you. I always had somebody's baby. I love other people's children. Still do.

Life is moving and I'm pretty happy. Then…

The Call

It was November 2010 the Monday before thanksgiving. My soon to be ex-husband called. Lain hey, what's going on? I'm hey I'm good nothing too much. What's up with you? Uh he says umm I need a favor… ok what you need? Can you go to the doctor with me tomorrow? Something is wrong and I'm not sure what. I know you understand all that terminology. I determined that it must be serious if he's calling me. So, the next day we go. We arrived at a small doctor's office on

Germantown avenue. His doctor was a nice lady. She said to me he has some sort of respiratory infection. I knew that because when we got in the car he was nasally, and I could smell the infection. I asked him what the smell was, and he said oh my god you smell that too!! Yes! I do smell that. (we didn't know it at the time be we were smelling cancer)

She said that she had been treating him for 3 weeks and nothing had changed. She said she had even given him the antibiotic they give to people with anthrax and he still was not better. Her suggestion to us was to go to the emergency room at Jefferson Hospital and don't leave until they tell us what's wrong. Whoa! Wait I'm busy. Now now I have come to this visit but hours in the emergency room. I don't know about that. At least that's what I thought in my head. He looked and me and I agreed to go. We left the doctor's office both quiet and thinking. Then I said to him I can't go tonight it's Tuesday. My group meets tonight. It's because of you I started this group. I can't miss it. We had been going strong at that point for 7months. I will meet you in the morning and we can go then. I go to my meeting that night and share what had happened. The women were like whoa, what are you going to do? I had already made my decision that I was going to go. Boy oh boy did I get an ear full. Half the women were like noooo way noooo how! The other half were life well if it wasn't for him we wouldn't be here so go. I had already decided I was going.

The Diagnosis

We arrived at Jefferson, parked and walked in. It felt weird it was almost like we knew it was going to be bad. We were laughing and talking joking having a decent time. Yup in the emergency room. It was like we were friends again, best friends. One friend supporting another and guess what it was ok. No one in the world mattered in those hours. They were doing tests, asking questions, poking prodding and x-raying. They even did and HIV and aids test. They asked me to leave while they read him the results. When I came back in he had his head in his hands. I'm like what what what did they say. He like siiikkkkeee. I said booooyyy you Beda stop playing. We had a good laugh and kept talking killing time waiting for the results of the test to come back. Finally, 12 hours later. Sir you have cancer. Huh say that again yes sir you can Nasopharyngeal cancer. His head went down, and I hugged him. That is all I could do. I felt helpless. Now its Weds, the weds before thanksgiving. I stay with him that night it was truly a silent night. I was there but I don't think he realized I was there he was some place in his mind thinking. He said a few things about if he died. I assured him no one was dying. I went home thanksgiving morning. His family had planned on spending time with him and considering we were divorcing. I didn't want to stay around for that. I went to my home packed up my 13-year-old daughter and she and I came back to the house. I explained that daddy was sick, and we needed to see about him. Somewhere in my mind I had already resolved that I was going to be there for him. He was the father of my children and I knew I would not be ok if someone called me and told me that he had died.

The Living Diary of the Mad Black Woman

Tyler Perry surely wrote the story, but I lived that life for real. The only difference is I wasn't mad. I had an assignment, and I fulfilled it.

I left my home, the home I purchased and now I am back to the marital home we built together. It was uncomfortable, but I wasn't there to be comfortable. The doctors immediately set up follow up with a Jefferson doctor. Here we go do this rabbit hole again.

This doctor was the worst. His bedside manner, he had no empathy at all. He said Sir after reviewing all your test. You have stage 4 Nasopharyngeal Cancer. If you do nothing you have about 6 months to live. With treatment you will probably live 15 months. I thought I was going to throw up. The doctor was very matter of factly, quite nonchalant for dishing out a death sentence. He asked what my wife did something holistic for her heart, can I do the same thing. Why did he ask that? The next thing out of this doctor's mouth was nooooo! What! I had a buddy that tried to do natural therapy with no hesitation in his words he is like he's dead. If you go that route you will be dead too! Wow, I don't like this guy. Umm let's leave, wait honey he is still talking. So, what! I said, he can't tag your toe, he ain't God, well he maybe God to someone else but not us. I think he thought he was God to at least himself. We out! We left. I called our pcp the next day the doctor we been going to since my son was 2. He knows us. He sent us to Temple. That was bad too but not as bad. You could feel the empathy there. We saw 5 or 6 doctors. We saw the oncologist, radiation oncologist, ear, nose and throat doctor, nutritionist and social worker. By the time all of them left we were literally balled up on the floor crying together. It was horrible, the expectations. The side effects of chemotherapy my God noooo! It was terrible. Radiation uh uh no way. We are going the other way. Get us out of here. We asked for time to think it over. They tried to rush us to a decision, but we didn't let them. We told them don't call us we'll call you!

Home we went, the mood was sad. This load was heavy. How in the world are we going to get through this? He went to bed, very depressed and I went to the internet. What did other people do? Is there a holistic remedy for stage 4 cancer? Can we conquer this mountain alone?

Research! Research! Research!

So, it begins.... Where do I start? GOOGLE!! People who resolved cancer with holistic remedies. Does that exist? Why yes, yes it does. Go to Netflix and watch these movies

Food, Inc., Food Matters, Forks over knives, The Beautiful Truth there it is again, I heard it in Food Matter too but now this person is saying it again. The Gerson Therapy! What is this therapy these movies are referring to? I don't know but let's google it. "Gerson Therapy" oh there is a movie. "The Gerson Miracle" ok let's go watch it. Very interesting! This one sounds like the winner. This is the one! Time to do my happy dance! Lord if this is the direction we should go. Please let me understand it! We need to save his life. I don't want my children to have to bury their father. Oh! wait what? Why am I doing this again. Umm hello God why in the world did I get this assignment? He said he didn't want to be married to me. Why do I feel compelled to do this? You were raised right. I don't know, welp here goes everything!!

The Gerson Therapy

The Gerson Therapy what is this therapy. How does it work?

The Gerson® Therapy is a natural treatment that activates the body's extraordinary ability to heal itself through an organic, plant-based diet, raw juices, coffee enemas and natural supplements.

With its whole-body approach to healing, the Gerson Therapy naturally reactivates your body's magnificent ability to heal itself – with no damaging side effects. This a powerful, natural treatment boosts the body's own immune system to heal cancer, arthritis, heart disease, allergies, and many other degenerative diseases. Dr. Max Gerson developed the Gerson Therapy in the 1930s, initially as a treatment for his own debilitating migraines, and eventually as a treatment for degenerative diseases such as skin tuberculosis, diabetes and, most famously, cancer.

Tell the Family

We told the family one by one what was happening. I think in retrospect we could have skipped some of them. It was hard for them to handle. I told my mother. She said ok, and that her and my dad would support my decision. She spoke way to soon. My dad called me and just asked one question, Why? My response was I am the woman that you raised. Silence and then click. Let's just say daddy wasn't happy with some of the things my husband had done in the past.

He was happy I was going to get a do-over. Do-over delayed!

We explained the treatment that he had chosen. They pretty much didn't understand it. It would take some time, but they would understand it shortly. We explained how labor intensive it would be. We counted the cost of groceries. Everybody got in it. We started! Whew! This is hard.

Everybody donated time, energy and money! Lots of money. We had people bringing cash, food stamps, and fruit and vegetables donation. It was truly a kalaka effort.

The following is the schedule:

Daily Schedule – Coffee break mean a coffee enema, not have a cup of coffee.

AM Morning

7:00 Rise and shine

7:15 Coffee Break (Be sure to eat a bite of fruit before enema)

7:45

1) Start oatmeal and coffee concentrate

2) Make citrus juice (Lugol's and potassium)

3) Sort medications for the day

8:00 Eat breakfast (orange juice and meds)

8:30

1) Wash the vegetables and fruits that you will use for the day's juices and meals

2) Strain the coffee

3) Start the Special soup (Hippocrates)

9:00 Green juice (potassium)

9:30 Carrot-Apple juice (Lugol's and potassium

10:00 Carrot apple juice – potassium and lugols solution

11:00 Carrot juice (2 Liver tablets) Prepare potatoes and vegetables for lunch

11:15 Coffee Break

PM Afternoon/Evening

12:00

1) Green juice (potassium)

2) Prepare lunch Salad Start vegetables and watch that they do not burn

1:00 Special (Hippocrates) soup Eat lunch

2:00 Green juice (potassium)

3:00 Carrot juice (w/2 Liver tablets)

4:00 Coffee Break + Carrot juice (w/Liver tablets)

5:00 Carrot-Apple juice (2 Liver tablets)

6:00 Green juice (potassium) Prepare dinner, salad, potatoes, vegetables, carrot-apple juice, etc.   7:00 Eat dinner, carrot and apple juice and meds

8:00 Coffee Break Put together a fruit plate to nibble on through the night

10:00 Coffee Break (Be sure to eat some fruit first)

AM Late Night/Early Morning

3:00 Coffee Break, if ordered by physician. (Eat first)

We did this every day! Day in and day out! We tried other things too! We added Pau D'Arco tea. Flaxseed oil mixed with yogurt, essiac tea. Oh, my goodness Essiac tea. So many benefits but when I say taste terrible. It tastes straight like dirt. Just plain ol' nasty! He drank it and so did I. We went vegan cold turkey! No plans, no prep just we vegan now. No one was allowed to bring outside food in the house. If anyone had a problem or was angry was not allowed in the house either. It needed to be calm and peaceful. Then it was decided after 5 months maybe we should go to the Gerson clinic to make sure we were facilitating it correctly. He did not want to go to Mexico or Hungary. We went to a place in Hawaii. It was pretty nice we met some amazing people. Some I am still friends with til this day. It was some experience. It was the longest 2 weeks. No cheating on diets and that place. It was peaceful, no tv, no radio just nature all around. The ocean was right there. We went right after a tsunami had hit Japan. It has damaged a good amount of the island too. A lot of the hotels and resorts were closed for damage. I am probably the only person that has been to Hawaii and did not see Hawaii. We stayed in Hilo. I was there to learn. Head down, pay attention it's going to mean his life. So, I did just that. I became good friend with the chef. She was so nice. She was patient when teaching me. There were at least 10 people at the house. Not too many were in the kitchen with me. I am so thankful for this time. I learned so much.

Ok, back home we go after 2 weeks. We are right back at it. We found a doctor who worked as a Naturo pathic doctor and a Doctor of Osteopathic medicine. He was a God send. He knew when we needed to do anything holistic and when we needed to do something traditional. There is where I met an amazing nurse name Asia. She made our visits there for high dose vitamin c therapy in her words delicious. She was a pleasant personality. She became very fond of us. She visited us at the house and at the hospital that was way out of her way. That was way beyond the call of duty.

I can tell you when Dr. Lipton said do something holistic we did it. When he said do something traditional we did it. When he saw the Gerson list of what we did. He said he knew about it but was not aware how labor intensive it was. He was amazed at how long we had been doing this therapy. He was a good fit to this wellness journey. Dr. Lipton asked me to let up a bit and let him have some chips.

We were well on our way and then…….

Integration – Integrative Medicine

Integrative Medicine is the use traditional and natural medicine together to make an impact on the health of an individual.

Note: Every individual is unique and integration is determined by the needs of the individual. Integration is determined by the stage or progression of the disease.

The tumor was in his nose and throat. The part we could see was shrinking but the part we couldn't behind his nose wasn't shrinking fast.

Our naturopath suggested low dose chemotherapy and a round of radiation therapy. He said that we are winning holistically but we need to move faster. So, we added that therapy as suggested.

Working with the body naturally can be slow. His cancer was stage 4. The tumor behind his nose was pushing into his brain stem and had invaded his facial nerve. Dr. Lipton suggested the traditional therapy to give us an edge to continue working holistically.

It was hard to say yes. We had been working so diligently. We continued the diet and took a break from the herbs and the coffee enemas while he took the traditional treatment. His body was so strong from all the holistic work we had been doing that he didn't get sick or lose his hair. 3 doses of chemo and radiation therapy. Scary but done. It gave us time we needed to get back to the therapy. High dose vitamin c therapy with glutathione to boost the immune system.

After all this work he is looking good!! Wow, Wow, and wow! We are so thankful.

Resolved!

You can't say cured in the United States. Since I am not a doctor I can't say I cured anything. However, after 9 months of hard intensive work and now the words we were waiting to hear. There is no more cancer in your body. We heard those words Aug 11, 2011. It is now 2017 he is still cancer free and has never had not one reoccurrence. What we know about cancer is in most cases, not all. It comes back once, twice and usually the second or the third time it takes the person out. We are all thankful that he is still alive to irk our lives!! Laugh out loud for real!!!

Darlaina Rose the Health Coach

Darlaina how can I heal myself? What can I do to get better? What can

I do for my high blood pressure, diabetes and poor eating habits? How can I gain weight? How can I lose weight? What can I do for my allergies? What can I do for my flu? Should I take the flu shot? What about grave disease? Crohn's disease? Question after question after question.

I did the research and answered each one of them. After a few years of this, I decided to become a health guru. I immersed myself in everything health and wellness. Mind, body and soul we are connected. How come some people get sick and others don't? I then decided to get a certification from Institute for Integrative Nutrition. I learned so much and continuing my education every day I learn something new. Life is amazing take care of yourself you only get once chance to live this life. The is the live show this is not dress rehearsal. Stay Grateful for this life and all that you get to do in it.

The House Guest and The Sister

I had a house guest come over. She was going to hang out with me for a while for work. When she arrived her blood, pressure was through the roof. She decided that she wasn't going to the hospital. I marched to kitchen and the first thing I gave her was Apple cider vinegar and baking soda together. I set the juicer up and right then I get a call. Hello sister, hey my blood pressure is up what can I do for it myself. I told her to do the apple cider vinegar and the baking soda. I told her to juice parsley, cucumber and celery. I told her to infuse her water with the same 3 ingredients and drink it overnight. I did the same thing for my house guest. After an hour both of their blood pressures were down remarkably. By morning almost simultaneously both of their blood pressures were normal. My house guest was so funny she called her husband and said "baby I'm never coming home Darlaina takes way better care of me than you." Wow we had a great laugh. As long as she stayed with me she ate better, she continued to infuse her water. She took the water to work and before you know it she had all her co-workers infusing their water. Some of them reached out and asked questions related to their own health concerns.

The Flu

Lady Rose Lady Rose please I feel terrible what can I do. My body hurts. This is an easy one. Get some fresh ginger cut it up, boil it and drink it. You can add a little honey to it. Grab some echinacea and golden seal take according to the package and call me in the morning. A few days later.... Thank you Lady Rose I am so much better. You can cut days off this illness by doing this.

Headaches

Mommy I have a headache! Ok daughter, grab some white willow bark and some peppermint oil. Take the white willow bark and then rub the peppermint oil on your temples and take a nap. Thank you, mommy I am good now.

Heart Disease

How can I get my heart stronger? Hawthorne Berry tea or capsules,

Coq10, Hibiscus tea or capsules.

Oh No Sister

My sister is ill. She had been in the hospital for over 30 days. She is waiting to get a procedure done. However, her hemoglobin is way too low. It's been so low the doctors are saying she needs a blood transfusion. As a Jehovah's Witness that is not happening. After visiting her learning, the problem, I went home to research. I researched natural ways to raise hemoglobin. I learned that certain foods block iron absorption. I find out what she needed and take it all to the hospital. The foods that block iron absorption: tomatoes, almonds, chocolate and caffeine. When I arrived at the hospital, guess what was on her plate? Tomato salad, black coffee, chocolate cake and somebody gave her a big can of Almonds! Ugh all this food is counter acting all the work they are doing. It unfortunate that the doctors don't know. According to my research doctors only get about 10 hours of nutritional training during all those years of training. I had read somewhere about a pharmaceutical company attempting to reduce those hours to 5 saying that the 10 hours are excessive. Wow really, excessive hearing this makes no common sense at all. As far as I know it's still 10 hours. I brought my sister a list of foods she could eat and the foods she could not eat. I brought her a basket of fruits that she could have along with a bottle of liquid gold. It was black nasty gold, but it would save her from any more unfruitful days. It was black strap molasses. I told her to take 2 tablespoons two times a day. In a matter of days her hemoglobin went from a 6 to a 12. She was then able to get her treatment and leave the hospital. Done and done.

Anemia in my friends

One of my friends was complaining that she was so tired all the time. She said her days had to be shortened most of the time because she was tired. When I inquired why she said she was anemic. She said that she had been taking iron, but she remained energy less. I said oh well just try the black strap molasses. It doesn't taste good, but it worked for my sister. I left her with that information. A few days later she told me she got it. She was elated she said she had more energy than she ever had. She could clean her home and take care of her mom. She just said it tasted so bad. I told her to try it with a chaser. Drink orange juice after taking it. She still takes it to this day. I have given this remedy to many with great results. One of my friends after having weight loss surgery suffered iron deficiency. I told her to try the black strap molasses. She said it tastes so bad. She found capsules. She reported her iron had increased to normal levels and continues to take the remedy to this day.

How can I help you?

Do you need to lose belly fat? Are you suffering from hypertension or diabetes? Do you need a weight loss plan? Here a few tips enjoy!! If you are interested in consulting with me don't hesitate to reach out.

www.DarlainaRose.com

Facebook, Twitter and Instagram "Darlaina Rose"

I live in a spirit of gratitude always. If you would like to receive your gratitude rock. (small shipping and handling fee) Email us at info@darlainarose.com

Note: Darlaina Rose is a Natural Health Professional and her studies have included body systems, Herbs and natural nutrition.

As a Natural Health Professional, she teaches about natural health maintenance giving clients consultations pertaining to the natural means by which they can have a healthier lifestyle. She deals strictly in helping people to improve their general health and fitness through better nutrition; improved lifestyle and health habits; and positive mental attitudes. Darlaina Rose is NOT a Medical Doctor and cannot legally diagnose diseases, prescribe drugs or recommend treatments for specific disease conditions and that he/she will not perform any functions of a licenses field.

Lower Your Blood Pressure

Juice cucumber, celery and parsley can use these same ingredients to infuse your water

Diabetes

Eat Raw, raw meaning most of your food not cooked. Raw, whole foods, one ingredients.

Watch the movie Raw for 30 days for details

Heart Disease

Coenzyme Q10, Omega-3 Fatty Acids, Green Tea, Pomegranate, Magnesium and Potassium

Lose Belly Fat

Add Cayenne, seaweed and green tea to your diet, add abdominal exercises, HIIT exercises, drink water, get enough sleep, no processed foods, reduce stress

Final thought: I believe that everything we need to heal our bodies is here. God has given us everything we need to heal ourselves naturally.

Hippocrates said, "let thy food by thy medicine and thy medicine thy food"

I am in no way against doctors and hospitals. They provide us with much needed services. I believe if you help the doctors to help you, you will live a very long life. Be committed to eating better, exercising, prayer and meditation. We are all connected mind body and soul. We are fearfully and wonderfully made. Take time out to take care of this one body that you get. Care you it and it will care for you.

You can be, do or have anything you want in this world. All you have to do is Ask, for it, believe you will receive it, (that means work for it) and wait to receive it. Here is a writing that was given to me in 2008 and I always kept it close to me. I now share it with you. I know that for sure you are enough to accomplish anything you put your mind to.

"I am Enough"

Today, I am enough.

I am smart enough.

Wise Enough.

Clever Enough.

Resourceful Enough.

Able Enough

Confident Enough.

I am connected to enough People to accomplish my Heart's desire.

I have enough to pull of Magic and Miracles.

Enough is all I Need.

Enough is What I have.

I have more than Enough!

As I do all that I can do, I'm able to do more and more.

I am excited to be alive, I rejoice and re-choice every day to make my life better.

I am happy, healthy prosperous, successful, rich, loving, loved and beloved.

I am comfortable with myself, so I am comfortable with all others.

I confidently greet each day with a smile on my face and love in my heart.

Everyone who meets me is warmed by the radiance of my attitude.

I work on my attitude continuously. I read positive, inspiring, and uplifting books.

I listen to audiotapes and CDs during my driving and exercise times.

I associate with friendly, caring, nurturing people who are involved doing important things.

The people with whom I associated want more for me that I want for myself.

The projects with which I am involved WOW my soul.

I am passionately on-purpose to do good, be good, and help others to do the same.

I am enough, I have enough, I do enough.

I am Enough!

-Unknown

10 Things to do today for better Health

1. *Drink Water – at least 8, 8oz glasses per day.*

2. *Sleep More – you need your rest. Determine how many hours of sleep you need to feel refreshed.*

3. *Exercise – 15 minutes a day to start. Walking around the block, up and down your stairs even jumping rope.*

4. *Practice Gratitude, write down what you are grateful for.*

5. *Add Sea salt to your water. The salt will aid with absorption as well as provide essential trace minerals.*

6. *Eat more Green leafy vegetables. Kale, chard, spinach etc.*

7. *Eat dark chocolate – at least 70% cocao its good for your heart*

8. *Meditate*

9. *Have a meatless Monday*

10. *Take a multi-vitamin multi-mineral*

Health   Planner

Use this planner for the next 30 days to keep track of your Health and wellness goals.

By

Darlaina Rose

HEALTH MONTHLY GOALS

1._____

2._____

3._____

4._____

5._____

HOW I WILL ACHIEVE THESE GOALS

_____

_____

BAD HABITS TO BREAK / GOOD HABITS TO MAKE

1._____

2._____

3._____

4._____

Notes

_____

_____

_____

_____

_____

_____

_____

MONTHLY CHECK IN

Measurement

Weight_____ Right Arm _____Left Arm_____

Chest_____ Waist_____ Hips_____ Right

Thigh_____ Left Thigh_____ Gain / Loss_____

lbs. _____ Inches_____

NOTES

_____

_____

_____

_____

_____

_____

_____

_____

Day 1 Date: _____

THOUGHTS

_____
_____
_____
_____

MENU

*Breakfast*_____

*Lunch*_____

*Dinner*_____

*Snacks*_____

EXERCISE

_____
_____
_____
_____
_____
_____

SHOPPING LIST / NOTES

Day 2 Date: _____

THOUGHTS

_____

_____

_____

_____

MENU

*Breakfast*_____

*Lunch*_____

*Dinner*_____

*Snacks*_____

EXERCISE

_____

_____

_____

_____

_____

_____

_____

SHOPPING LIST / NOTES

Day3 Date: _____

THOUGHTS

_____
_____
_____
_____

MENU

*Breakfast*_____

*Lunch*_____

*Dinner*_____

*Snacks*_____

EXERCISE

_____
_____
_____
_____
_____
_____
_____

SHOPPING LIST / NOTES

Day 4 Date: _____

THOUGHTS

_____
_____
_____
_____

MENU

*Breakfast*_____

*Lunch*_____

*Dinner*_____

*Snacks*_____

EXERCISE

_____
_____
_____
_____
_____
_____
_____

SHOPPING LIST / NOTES

HEALTH MONTHLY GOALS

1._____

2._____

3._____

4._____

5._____

HOW I WILL ACHIEVE THESE GOALS

_____

_____

BAD HABITS TO BREAK / GOOD HABITS TO MAKE

1._____

2._____

3._____

4._____

Notes

_____

_____

_____

MONTHLY CHECK IN

Measurement

Weight_____ Right Arm _____Left Arm_____
Chest_____ Waist_____ Hips_____ Right
Thigh_____ Left Thigh_____ Gain / Loss_____
lbs. _____ Inches_____

NOTES

_____
_____
_____
_____
_____
_____
_____
_____
_____
_____
_____
_____
_____
_____
_____
_____
_____
_____
_____
_____

THOUGHTS

_____
_____
_____
_____

MENU

*Breakfast*_____

*Lunch*_____

*Dinner*_____

*Snacks*_____

EXERCISE

_____
_____
_____
_____
_____
_____
_____

SHOPPING LIST / NOTES

HEALTH MONTHLY GOALS

1._____

2._____

3._____

4._____

5._____

HOW I WILL ACHIEVE THESE GOALS

_____

_____

BAD HABITS TO BREAK / GOOD HABITS TO MAKE

1._____

2._____

3._____

4._____

Notes

_____

_____

_____

MONTHLY CHECK IN

Measurement

Weight_____ Right Arm _____Left Arm_____
Chest_____ Waist_____ Hips_____ Right
Thigh_____ Left Thigh_____ Gain / Loss_____
lbs. _____ Inches_____

NOTES

_____
_____
_____
_____
_____
_____
_____
_____
_____
_____
_____
_____
_____
_____
_____
_____
_____
_____
_____
_____

THOUGHTS

_____

_____

_____

_____

MENU

Breakfast_____

Lunch_____

Dinner_____

Snacks_____

EXERCISE

_____

_____

_____

_____

_____

_____

_____

SHOPPING LIST / NOTES

Day 5 Date: _____

THOUGHTS

_____
_____
_____
_____

MENU

*Breakfast*_____

*Lunch*_____

*Dinner*_____

*Snacks*_____

EXERCISE

_____
_____
_____
_____
_____
_____
_____

SHOPPING LIST / NOTES

Day 6 Date: _____

THOUGHTS

_____

_____

_____

_____

MENU

*Breakfast*_____

*Lunch*_____

*Dinner*_____

*Snacks*_____

EXERCISE

_____

_____

_____

_____

_____

_____

_____

SHOPPING LIST / NOTES

_____
_____
_____
_____
_____
_____
_____
_____
_____
_____
_____
_____
_____
_____
_____
_____
_____
_____
_____
_____
_____
_____
_____
_____
_____
_____
_____
_____
_____
_____

Day 7 Date: _____

THOUGHTS

_____
_____
_____
_____

MENU

*Breakfast*_____

*Lunch*_____

*Dinner*_____

*Snacks*_____

EXERCISE

_____
_____
_____
_____
_____
_____

SHOPPING LIST / NOTES

Day 8 Date: _____

THOUGHTS

_____
_____
_____
_____

MENU

*Breakfast*_____

*Lunch*_____

*Dinner*_____

*Snacks*_____

EXERCISE

_____
_____
_____
_____
_____
_____

SHOPPING LIST / NOTES

Day 9 Date: _____

THOUGHTS

_____

_____

_____

_____

MENU

Breakfast_____

Lunch_____

Dinner_____

Snacks_____

EXERCISE

_____

_____

_____

_____

_____

_____

_____

SHOPPING LIST / NOTES

Day 10 Date: _____

THOUGHTS

_____
_____
_____
_____

MENU

*Breakfast*_____

*Lunch*_____

*Dinner*_____

*Snacks*_____

EXERCISE

_____
_____
_____
_____
_____
_____

SHOPPING LIST / NOTES

Day 11 Date: _____

THOUGHTS

_____
_____
_____
_____

MENU

*Breakfast*_____

*Lunch*_____

*Dinner*_____

*Snacks*_____

EXERCISE

_____
_____
_____
_____
_____
_____

78

SHOPPING LIST / NOTES

Day 12 Date: _____

THOUGHTS

_____
_____
_____
_____

MENU

*Breakfast*_____

*Lunch*_____

*Dinner*_____

*Snacks*_____

EXERCISE

_____
_____
_____
_____
_____
_____
_____

SHOPPING LIST / NOTES

Day 13 Date: _____

THOUGHTS

_____

_____

_____

_____

MENU

Breakfast_____

Lunch_____

Dinner_____

Snacks_____

EXERCISE

_____

_____

_____

_____

_____

_____

_____

SHOPPING LIST / NOTES

Day 14 Date: _____

THOUGHTS

_____

_____

_____

_____

MENU

*Breakfast*_____

*Lunch*_____

*Dinner*_____

*Snacks*_____

EXERCISE

_____

_____

_____

_____

_____

_____

_____

SHOPPING LIST / NOTES

Day 15 Date: _____

THOUGHTS

_____
_____
_____
_____

MENU

Breakfast_____

Lunch_____

Dinner_____

Snacks_____

EXERCISE

_____
_____
_____
_____
_____
_____

SHOPPING LIST / NOTES

Day 16 Date: _____

THOUGHTS

_____
_____
_____
_____

MENU

*Breakfast*_____

*Lunch*_____

*Dinner*_____

*Snacks*_____

EXERCISE

_____
_____
_____
_____
_____
_____

SHOPPING LIST / NOTES

Day 17 Date: _____

THOUGHTS

_____
_____
_____
_____

MENU

*Breakfast*_____

*Lunch*_____

*Dinner*_____

*Snacks*_____

EXERCISE

_____
_____
_____
_____
_____
_____

SHOPPING LIST / NOTES

Day 18 Date: _____

THOUGHTS

_____

_____

_____

_____

MENU

*Breakfast*_____

*Lunch*_____

*Dinner*_____

*Snacks*_____

EXERCISE

_____

_____

_____

_____

_____

_____

_____

SHOPPING LIST / NOTES

Day 19 Date: _____

THOUGHTS

_____
_____
_____
_____

MENU

*Breakfast*_____

*Lunch*_____

*Dinner*_____

*Snacks*_____

EXERCISE

_____
_____
_____
_____
_____
_____
_____

SHOPPING LIST / NOTES

Day 20 Date: _____

THOUGHTS

_____
_____
_____
_____

MENU

*Breakfast*_____

*Lunch*_____

*Dinner*_____

*Snacks*_____

EXERCISE

_____
_____
_____
_____
_____
_____

SHOPPING LIST / NOTES

Day 21 Date: _____

THOUGHTS

_____
_____
_____
_____

MENU

*Breakfast*_____

*Lunch*_____

*Dinner*_____

*Snacks*_____

EXERCISE

_____
_____
_____
_____
_____
_____

SHOPPING LIST / NOTES

Day 22 Date: _____

THOUGHTS

_____
_____
_____
_____

MENU

*Breakfast*_____

*Lunch*_____

*Dinner*_____

*Snacks*_____

EXERCISE

_____
_____
_____
_____
_____
_____
_____

SHOPPING LIST / NOTES

Day 23 Date: _____

THOUGHTS

_____

_____

_____

_____

MENU

*Breakfast*_____

*Lunch*_____

*Dinner*_____

*Snacks*_____

EXERCISE

_____

_____

_____

_____

_____

_____

SHOPPING LIST / NOTES

Day 24 Date: _____

THOUGHTS

_____
_____
_____
_____

MENU

*Breakfast*_____

*Lunch*_____

*Dinner*_____

*Snacks*_____

EXERCISE

_____
_____
_____
_____
_____
_____

SHOPPING LIST / NOTES

Day 25 Date: _____

THOUGHTS

_____

_____

_____

_____

MENU

*Breakfast*_____

*Lunch*_____

*Dinner*_____

*Snacks*_____

EXERCISE

_____

_____

_____

_____

_____

_____

_____

SHOPPING LIST / NOTES

Day 26 Date: _____

THOUGHTS

_____
_____
_____
_____

MENU

*Breakfast*_____

*Lunch*_____

*Dinner*_____

*Snacks*_____

EXERCISE

_____
_____
_____
_____
_____
_____

SHOPPING LIST / NOTES

Day 27 Date: _____

THOUGHTS

_____

_____

_____

_____

MENU

*Breakfast*_____

*Lunch*_____

*Dinner*_____

*Snacks*_____

EXERCISE

_____

_____

_____

_____

_____

_____

_____

SHOPPING LIST / NOTES

Day 28 Date: _____

THOUGHTS

_____

_____

_____

_____

MENU

*Breakfast*_____

*Lunch*_____

*Dinner*_____

*Snacks*_____

EXERCISE

_____

_____

_____

_____

_____

_____

SHOPPING LIST / NOTES

Day 29 Date: _____

THOUGHTS

_____

_____

_____

_____

MENU

*Breakfast*_____

*Lunch*_____

*Dinner*_____

*Snacks*_____

EXERCISE

_____

_____

_____

_____

_____

_____

_____

SHOPPING LIST / NOTES

Day 30 Date: _____

THOUGHTS

_____
_____
_____
_____

MENU

*Breakfast*_____

*Lunch*_____

*Dinner*_____

*Snacks*_____

EXERCISE

_____
_____
_____
_____
_____
_____

SHOPPING LIST / NOTES

Testimonials

It's a beautiful feeling to have your very own health coach! You can see it in my eyes, my body and I FEEL wonderful! God knows best and he blessed me with Darlaina Rose. Go get your blessing and hit her up! - *Phoebe M. Grimes -Optum Atlanta Ga*

I didn't even know there was a such thing as a sitting disease. Thanks to you I am up and walking around during my work hours. – *Rob Williams, Freelance Photographer Atlanta, Ga*

Thank You D.Rose, for all you do on the Life Changes Alliances platform. You gave me much clarity on previous health changes I made. Thank you so much Your Awesome. *-Desmond "Big D" Desmond, LCA*

Darlaina Rose my mom is clean and sober from pepsi! Woohoo! - *Sabrina "Bri Bri" Black, LCA*

Thank you so much for the blood pressure reducing juice remedy. My blood pressure was normal by morning! – *Mattie Harrigan, Employment Coach*

In my life, I've had the opportunity to meet strong, smart, independent women from every walk of life. They've inspired me in many ways, and continue to remind me that women are connected by many common threads. Darlaina in has inspired me to be fearless and to walk by faith and not by sight. She's inspired me to continue to set goals and conquer my fears.

The sky is not even the limit for what God has for Darlaina. *-Gwen Dillard – Temple University Hospital*

I am so proud of Darlaina Rose for taking her compassion for life and sharing it with us all. Her determination for assisting all to have a better quality of life is amazing. *-Sharlene Waller, Chief of Staff for Isabella Fitzerald*

You inspire me by your motivation, by your words they leave a lasting impression, by the example of your life. *Sequille Boldon-United States Navy*

Girl you are the bomb! You always know the right thing to say at the Perfect time. You give the right encouragement to help others to Keep It Moving – *Yvette Gay-Jenkins,DCMH,*

You inspire me to always look and feel young. You inspire me to climb any mountain that stand before me no matter how big or small. You always inspire me to start out fresh everyday in reaching my goals. To never give up and to give it all that I got and then some…even when it looks like its just not working out…to keep moving toward my goal and building upon it 'til I've accomplished what I set out to do. It's easy to quit but rewarding to press to the end. *–Bettina Nesbitt, BAS*

www.DarlainaRose.com   Twitter @darlainarose

Facebook Darlaina Rose   Like my Page at
www.FaceBook.com/RoseWellnessGroup

Use your 30 day Health Planner Included Inside!

Get your 10 things to do for your health today list inside!

www.ingramcontent.com/pod-product-compliance
Lightning Source LLC
Chambersburg PA
CBHW070253290326
41930CB00041B/2483